ABORTION
THE FACTS

ABORTION

THE FACTS

MICHAEL JAMES SCOTT

Darton, Longman & Todd

First published in Great Britain in 1973 by
Darton, Longman & Todd Ltd
85 Gloucester Road, London SW7 4SU

ISBN 0 232, 51253 1

Revised and reprinted, 1974

Printed in Great Britain by

The Markham Press of Kingston Ltd
Surbiton, Surrey.

Contents

Colour Illustrations

(between pages 32 and 33)

1) Human Life at Eight Weeks
2) Suction Abortion at 10 Weeks
3) D & C Abortion at 12 Weeks
4) Salt Poisoning Abortion at 19 Weeks

With permission, *Handbook on Abortion,* Willke, Hiltz and Hayes, Publishing Co., Inc., Cincinatti, Ohio.

Chapter One

The 1967 Abortion Act

In 1803 abortion became an offence from the time of conception. The law was changed in 1861 under the Offences against
the Person Act, which laid down that an abortion whenever induced was a felony punishable by life imprisonment. In 1929
the Infant Life (Preservation) Act amended the law to say that
abortion would no longer be regarded as a felony if carried out
in good faith for the sole purpose of preserving the life of the
mother. The Bourne case in 1938 was the next move towards a
liberalised abortion law. Mr. Aleck Bourne, a London gynaecologist, publicly performed an abortion on a 14 year-old girl who
had been raped by two soldiers. He was subsequently tried, and
the judge, Judge Macnaughten, liberally interpreted the words
of the exceptions clause of the 1929 Act. Mr. Bourne was
acquitted. (It is interesting that he has since joined the ranks
of the anti-abortionists). Physicians took this to mean that they
were legally entitled to perform abortions, but how far they
could go without transgressing the law remained unclear.

The Abortion Law Reform Association (ALRA), was
formed in 1936 and devoted itself to the passage of a liberal
abortion law. It was behind the seven abortion bills that were
introduced into Parliament without success before David Steel
brought in his Bill in 1967. Until David Steel's abortion Act
was well under debate, there was no organised opposition to a
liberal abortion law. Finally SPUC, the Society for the Protection of Unborn Children, was formed. It was able to present a
petition with more than half a million signatories appealing
for a Royal Commission on abortion.

This followed the lead of the President of the Royal College
of Obstetricians and Gynaecologists who, in a letter to The
Times of 21 January 1966 made a public appeal for the setting

up of a special committee or commission to examine all facets of the law pertaining to terminating pregnancy before the terms of the new legislation was presented to Parliament. The RCOG unanimously adopted a report stating that the present situation (i.e. that existing from 1929 onwards) 'commends itself to most gynaecologists'. In the RCOG report to the Lane Commission they write, 'Whilst the Bill was under discussion the legislators were repeatedly warned of the implications and outcome of what they proposed. The warnings were given verbally by Officers of this College and published with constructive guidance to the legislators.' Their advice 'was in certain important respects disregarded, but subsequent events have shown how fully justified were our forebodings.' Psychiatric opinion tended to be more liberal than that of gynaecologists.

The proponents of the Bill went to great length to assure everyone that it was not abortion on demand that was being legalised. They spoke instead of the 'hard' cases, the women with six children, the raped schoolgirl, the deaths from back-street abortions, the astronomical number of illegal abortions. The figure of 100,000 illegal abortions a year was often quoted, and came to be commonly accepted. On 15 July 1967, after 27 hours continuous debate, the Bill passed through the Commons by 167 votes to 83. From there it went to the Lords, on 27 October 1967 it received the Royal Assent, and on 27 April 1968 it became law.

Under the provisions of the Act, abortion by a registered medical practitioner is permitted, if two medical practitioners form the opinion 'in good faith' that either:

a) the continuance of the pregnancy would involve risk to the life of the pregnant woman or of injury to the physical or mental health of the pregnant women, or any existing children of her family, greater than if the pregnancy were terminated.

b) that there is substantial risk that if the child were born it would suffer from such physical or mental abnormalities as to be seriously handicapped.

The Act also provided that, in determining whether the continuance of a pregnancy would involve risk of injury to health, account may be taken of the pregnant woman's 'actual or reasonably forseeable environment'.

Section 4 of the Act provided that no one shall be under any duty to participate in any treatment authorised by the Act to which he has a conscientious objection.

Dr. Goodhart has commented, 'since the almost non-existent risk to the life of a healthy woman in an abortion properly performed early on in pregnancy is indeed likely to be less than the present very low, but not wholly negligible risk in childbirth, it is hard to see how any doctor could justify a refusal to give such a certificate. Whatever Parliament may have intended, this is in effect abortion on demand, subject only to a doctor's right to refuse to participate if he can prove a genuine conscientious objection'. [1] In practice, then, the Act could be used to permit abortion on demand.

In any case, most expectant women, owing to biochemical changes, experience considerable swings of mood and are sometimes depressed. The more severe anxieties could be held to bring the woman within the 'mental health' clause of the Act.

Special private clinics were licensed to deal with abortions, as the National Health Service could not hope to cope alone. The fee at these clinics would be anything from £50 to £200. There was no restriction put on foreign girls entering Britain for an abortion. No special facilities were made available in the NHS. It is not surprising, then, that within three years of the Act's becoming operative it proved possible to obtain the signature of 260 Members of Parliament to a motion calling for an investigation into all facets of the Act. The final outcome of this was that the Secretary of State for Social Services appointed Mrs. Justice Lane to head a committee of inquiry into the Act. However, the terms of reference of the Lane Committee were restricted to the working of the Act; they were not to consider revision of the grounds for legal abortion. The Lane Committee reported on April 3rd 1974 and but for racketeering largely condoned the present situation.

It seems paradoxical that, at a time when there has never been greater affluence, a greater means of preventing conception and greater tolerance of the unmarried mother, abortion should be made legal. In the last decade the purchasing power of the individual has gone up by 30%[2] . Little of the extra income has been spent on food. The big increase in spending has been on cars, alcoholic drink, entertainment, recreation and housing. Yet the problem seems to be that parents continually demand more and more as a minimum standard of life for themselves and for their children. Luxuries become conveniences and then necessities. Consequently, parents are increasingly unwilling to accept the cut in their own standard of life which the arrival of a new baby may mean. With an ever-lengthening list of wants, abortion is seen as a useful safeguard of material well-being.

The advent of the contraceptive pill has contributed to the pressure for legalised abortion. The woman taking the pill feels so sure that she will not conceive that she finds it psychologically traumatic if she does so. Abortion comes to be seen as a necessary back-up for failed contraceptives. That the former is a post-life and the latter a pre-life situation is usually glossed over. Rather, as surveys in Korea, Taiwan and elsewhere have shown, women who use contraceptives "are more likely than others to seek an abortion if they become pregnant, because of either contraceptive failure or discontinuation of use."[3]

Chapter Two

The Nature of the Unborn

To begin to consider the nature of the unborn child is immediately to run the risk of being labelled "anti-abortionist", and
consequently dismissed. Such was the fate of Niellson in Sweden, when he wrote *The Everyday Miracle*. This described the
nature of the unborn with accuracy, great beauty and some
remarkable pictures, even though it was not the purpose of
the book to consider the problem of abortion.

Yet those who will not seriously consider the nature of
what they would freely dispose of are surely at best guilty of
intellectual cowardice, at worst extreme callousness. By the
same token one must strongly criticise those who talk about
the unborn as if it were brought by the mythical stork, and
fail to take the mother into consideration.

Defining the meeting of sperm and ovum, Professor
Goodhart, of the Department of Zoology at Cambridge has
said: 'This is the point after, but not before which it becomes
capable of completing its development without any further
stimulus from outside. Once activated the organism will carry
on its development until it dies'.[4] Thus conception marks a
real biological discontinuity. The single cell formed at conception contains all the information, in the form of genes,
that will cause it to develop into a unique individual. The
fertilised egg (ovum) thus already contains all the instructions
which determine the future configuration of the body and the
face which will give it the 'family likeness' and the future
colour of the eyes, skin and hair. We have then at conception
a distinct entity which is never genetically identical with
either of its parents, but a blend of their gifts.

From the time of fusion of the sperm with the egg, the

fertilised ovum (conceptus) contains 46 thread-like structures known as chromosomes. These are arranged in pairs, one member of each pair having been derived from the father and the other from the mother. The cells of cats usually contain 88 chromosomes, those of mice 40 chromosomes. So whether a particular fertilised egg belongs to the human species can be indicated by the number of chromosomes it contains and the pattern of the chromosomes. It is not, however, a complete test, as a number of human abnormalities (such as mongolism) are associated with an abnormality in the number of chromosomes. Also other species, such as the marmoset, have the same number. However, it is a good indicator. From this brief survey of genetics it seems reasonable to conclude that we have at conception a genetically distinct individual which is of the human species.

Near the end of the first week the conceptus imbeds itself into the lining of the womb. This is called implantation. Implantation as such contributes nothing to the nature of the conceptus, it is merely the lodging of the conceptus in a convenient site so that it can be suitably nourished and have room to grow. The conceptus would develop equally well (to start with, at any rate) were it to implant in some other site such as the uterine tube or the peritoneal cavity.

About the time of implantation the conceptus, or more correctly the zygote, may divide, giving rise to two daughter cells, each of which may develop into one of a pair of so-called identical twins. In 4% of identical twins the splitting does not take place until well after implantation.[5]

The cells forming the embryo are separated from the maternal tissues by an outer shell of extra-embryonic cells. These give rise to the placenta and the protective membranes around the embryo. In this way the embryonic body is physically quite distinct from the mother, as well as having a different genetic make-up, and cannot be considered as part of the mother.

Geraldine Flanagan describes a baby of four weeks: "By the end of the first month a whole embryo is formed from head to heel, and is ¼ to ½ inch long. But the body has a head with rudimentary eyes, mouth and a brain that already shows some

14

human specialisation. There are a simple kidney, a liver, a digestive tract, a primitive umbilical cord and a blood stream and heart. The heart is usually beating by the 25th day.[6]

It appears, however, to have a tail and gill slits around its head. This had led some to think of the embryo as animal life that becomes human at a later stage of development. The alleged gills are not however openings, and have no gill fronds. It is actually tissue for the chin, cheeks and jaw. The apparent tail encloses the early spinal cord, which is temporarily longer than the rest of the body.

'In the 6th and 7th weeks', declares another authority, 'if the area of the lips is gently stroked the child responds by bending the upper body to one side and making a quick backward motion with his arms'.[7] Brain waves have been detected as early as 43 days.[8]

By the end of the third month the unborn child has become very active. He can now kick his legs, turn his feet, curl and fan his toes, make a fist, move his thumb, bend his wrist, turn his head, squint, frown, open his mouth and press his lips tightly together. Thumb sucking is also noted at this stage.[9] The fingernails appear, and he starts to urinate.[10] Children at this stage show genuine individual difference. Dr. Gessell, in his book *The Embryology of Behaviour,*[11] notes that:

'Our own repeated observation of foetal infants (an individual born and living at any time prior to 40 weeks gestation) left us with no doubt that psychologically they were individuals. Just as no two looked alike, so no two behaved alike. One was passive when another was alert. Even among the youngest there were discernible differences in vividness, reactivity and responsiveness. These were genuinely individual differences, already prophetic of the diversity which distinguishes the human family.'

In the fifth month (16-20 weeks) the unborn child becomes about one foot tall, and weighs approximately one pound. Hair begins to grow on his head and eyebrows, and a fringe of eyelashes appear. The child sleeps and wakes as he will after birth.[12] Each baby has a characteristic posture. Some always sleep with the chin resting on the chest, while others tilt the head back as far as it will go. He may sometimes be roused from sleep by external vibration.[13]

It is worth noting that not only the mother can be regarded as a patient, so also can the unborn child. About ten years ago, Dr. A.W. Liley, an obstetrician from New Zealand, performed an intra-uterine transfusion to treat an infant afflicted with RH disease. Since that time a number of other advances have been made, the most dramatic of which has been direct surgical operation on the unborn. Dr. Stanley Asensio, of the University of Puerto Rico School of Medicine, has actually taken the foetus out of the mother's womb, performed an operation, and then placed the foetus back into the womb, for it to be delivered later as a healthy normal child. The operation is so delicate that the surgeon must use fluid-filled gloves when handling the foetus. [14]

If a child is born prematurely at 20 weeks, it has a 10% or less chance of survival. The ability to survive outside the womb is termed "viability". As medical science advances, the younger the age at which a prematurely born child can be viewed as viable. It is possible that in the coming decade viability will be down to twelve weeks, or even earlier, given the development of an artificial placenta. The date of viability is a measure of the increasing sophistication of our external life-support systems.

It is difficult, then, to see why the date of viability should be invoked as the time before which life may be terminated and after which it is accorded the full protection of the law. The present abortion law, in keeping with the notion of viability, allows abortion up to the 28th week. This concept, it should be admitted, has no ethical significance, and to judge a particular being's right to life by it is quite unjustified. We are all "non-viable", taken out of our natural environment. If stripped naked and placed at the North Pole I too would be non-viable, just as the unborn child prematurely extracted from his mother's womb becomes so.

In the last three months the unborn child gains most of the weight he will have at birth and outgrows his home in the womb. In the seventh month the hair on the baby's head may grow long. In the eighth month he gains about two pounds, mostly in protective padding that will keep his body warm

16

after birth. (These last three months are also important because he gains many immunities at this time). Finally, at the end of the nine months, the child is born. Birth involves both the emergence from the mother's womb and the severing of the umbilical cord. It marks the beginning of the child's existence physically detached from the mother's body. The only change that occurs at birth is a change in the external life-support system of the child.

The baby is no different after birth than before, except that he has changed his method of feeding and his means of obtaining oxygen. Before birth nutrition and oxygen came from his mother, through the baby's umbilical cord. After birth oxygen is obtained through his own lungs, and nutrition, when he is mature enough, through his own stomach.

Life is a process of development that begins at conception. To say of that process at any stage that human life has now begun is an entirely arbitrary decision. Such a decision would not matter if the unborn could be judged non-human, but analysis shows that the unborn appears structurally the same as humans. Humanity, however, is attested not merely by structure, but also by personality and achievement. To be considered in any way human the unborn child must have a developing physical basis for the future exhibition of personality. In cases where this basis is absent we have a genetic monster; the destruction of such a monster could not be held to be an abortion. In the same way, at the other end of life we may have a man suffering complete destruction of his physical basis for the exhibition of personality, and existing as a "vegetable". It is not murder to allow him to die (nor incidentally is it euthanasia: euthanasia is a direct attempt to interrupt the ability of a person to sustain life, this distinction must not be blurred).

Personality has in some sense to be taken into account in our definition of humanity. However, to repeat a point made by D. Callahan, "to be human is not just to display here and now the full range of human characteristics. Human beings do not always think; sometimes they are asleep or drugged, or too young to think. Human beings are not always in relationships

17

with other, sometimes they are alone."[15] I do not forfeit my right to life merely because I am at present too tired to show my personality. Why then should the unborn forfeit his right because he is not at the moment showing his personality?

The American philosopher Ashley Montagu, in a letter to the New York Times, wrote that, 'humanity is an achievement, not an endowment.' In other words, man is not vested with human rights at creation, or at birth, or even as a 'newborn' child, but only much later when he contributes to the 'quality of life'. This achievement, according to Montagu, is the result of social interaction. Such a view of humanity has grave implications, not only for the unborn but also for many who have been born. The Nixons, Johnsons, Calleys and J. Edgar Hoovers of this world of power can all point to their social involvements to assert their claim to a humanity supposedly engendered by these involvements. Such involvement, however, is no help to the unborn foetus, who has yet to meet his mother, to the husband in a womb-like iron lung, or to the senile grandmother. Neither is that argument much help to the Helen Kellers, Ludwig von Beethovens, Friedrich Nietzsches and Lord Byrons, whose physical disabilities retard their social inter-actions.[16]

This philosophical by-product of the pro-abortionists will lead to a diminution of value and humanity accorded to the socially deprived among the born; the infant of six months, the spastic teenager, the adult in an iron lung, the lunatic in an asylum, the convicted criminal, the recluse, the hermit. It then seems possible that the practical as well as the logical distinctions will disappear among abortion, infanticide and the various sociological conveniences called 'mercy killing' to the detriment of the born as well as the unborn. It is worth noting that those who supported the 1967 Abortion Act went on to campaign for a euthanasia bill, and that two years ago such a bill was defeated in the House of Lords by only 61 votes to 40. Of 17 States in America which had legalised abortion, in seven there have already been persistent attempts to introduce euthanasia bills.

The recent pronouncement of the US Supreme Court was that not only was abortion permissible on demand up to the point of viability, but in the seventh, eighth and ninth months abortion was to be permitted for the sake of the health of the mother. The term "health" here was to be taken in the sense of the definition of the World Health Organisation: 'a state of complete physical, mental and social well-being, not simply the absence of illness and disease.' Never before in British or American Law has a baby in the last stages of pregnancy been so exposed to destruction at the desire of the parent.

Humanity viewed as an "achievement" the result of social interactions, cannot be accepted unless we are to countenance "a sociological disposal system, a dolce vita smoother and more antiseptic than any ever devised by any tyrant or Fuhrer"[17] It is worth pointing out that, even now, we are being asked to believe that "at birth the baby is only a potential human being,"[18] and can be regarded as disposable if it turns out to be, say, a spina-bifida baby. The principle of the sanctity of life is being eroded.

It is indeed strange that those who oppose abortion are labelled "reactionary", while those who support it are in fact supporting a highly elitist philosophy destined to preserve the adult establishment from being disturbed. What is more re-actionary than that?

Chapter Three

The Mother

As I have already noted, the passage of the 1967 Abortion Act was accompanied by frequent reference to the 'raped schoolgirl', or to the working class mother, worn out by constant child bearing and grossly abused by a continually drunk husband. It is ironic that even prior to the 1967 Act, abortion could probably be obtained on the NHS for such extreme cases. The reality of the present situation is different. Most abortions are totally unrelated to physical or mental health, and are demanded more readily and accepted more readily by the upper social classes. [19]

During the years 1970, 1971 and 1972, ten, nine and eight women respectively were treated under the clause which permits abortion in acute life-or-death situations. Figures of 36, 12 and 13 women are recorded for those allowed abortions on the grounds of grave injury to physical or mental health. Likelihood of severe physical or mental handicap of child was given as the justification in 1248, 2393 and 1175 cases. Yet during these same years the total number of abortions recorded was 86565, 126774 and 156741 respectively. The 'hard' cases thus form certainly no more than about 2% of abortions performed during that period.

Most abortions come under one of the following headings: neuroses, non-psychotic mental disorder, or transient situational disturbance. The figures for these for the year 1970 were respectively 46014, 19846 and 19175. For the year 1971 they were 73455, 24022 and 23944. These headings represent abortion on social or economic grounds. The headings cannot be regarded as serious psychiatric indications for abortion, for 'the psychiatrist when dealing with a non-psychotic patient is in an area without landmarks. [20]

One of the arguments of David Steel's Act was that abortion was relatively safe - yet, as Stallworthy noted: 'If termination of pregnancy were as safe as so many advocates of liberal abortion maintain, a patient suffering as a result of the operation could claim that professional negligence was responsible for her subsequent distress or disaster, and plead *res ipsa loquitur.* Such claims would generally be grossly unfair' [21] Stallworthy studied 1182 legal abortions performed in a teaching hospital. Nearly 17% of patients lost more than 500 mls of blood and 9.5% required a blood transfusion. Cervical lacerations occurred in 4.2% and the uterus was perforated in 1.2%.

Between January 1967 and December 1970, 1317 abortions were performed at the West Middlesex Hospital. The rate for serious complications was 16.8%. This figure included tearing of the cervix, injury to the bladder and bowel, perforation of the uterus. The rate was calculated leaving out those affected by urinary tract infection. The observations were only taken up to six weeks after termination. The long-term effects on the mothers can only be guessed. Certainly, 16.8% must be regarded as the absolute minimum complication rate.

On 1 March 1973 Dr. Margaret Wynn and Dr. Arthur Wynn, two distinguished sociologists, published a report [22] in which they carried out a detailed analysis of 75 recent medical publications on abortion from 12 countries. They reported that between 2 and 5% of women who had abortions became sterile as a result. Among those who became pregnant again as many as 30 to 40% had miscarriages, and the risk of other complications in early pregnancy amongst these women was doubled. The report also showed a 40% increase in premature births, with the consequent increased risk of the child being born deformed. At a press conference after the report was published, Dr. Arthur Wynn said that there could be 200 severely mentally handicapped children every year as a result of 150,000 abortions. He added: 'Abortion induced in young women, particularly prior to marriage, may be a cause of severe marital stress, subsequently leading to marital breakdown, separation and divorce.' [23]

The Wynn Report was generally regarded as an important piece of research. To quote one representative judgement, in a leading article the British Medical Journal said: 'The Wynns have produced a very serious indictment of legalised abortion which must be heeded by doctors and law-makers.'

On 3 March 1973, the day after this article appeared, Mr. Hull, Conservative MP for Wycombe, brought the Wynn report up. Questioning Sir Keith Joseph, Minister for Health and Social Services, Mr. Hull asked whether it was not time, in view of the Wynn's Report evidence, that the Government reviewed the Abortion Act and made sure abortions were limited to cases of medical necessity, and were not allowed as a means simply of saving embarrassment. In reply, Sir Keith spoke vaguely about certain shortcomings of the Wynn report, and said that it was necessary to wait for the Lane Committee's proposals. While the R.C.O.G. advised the Lane Committee that 'there is clear evidence that sequalae such as sterility, menorrhagea, recurrent abortion and premature labour are not uncommon amongst women who in youth had a pregnancy terminated' the Lane Report however speaks merely of possible risks and complications.

The psychological effect of abortion on the mother is the most difficult factor to elucidate. In 1966 the RCOG reported that "the incidence of serious permanent psychiatric aftermath from abortion is variously reported as being between 9 and 59%" It is often said guilt following an abortion is the result of Christian ethics. Yet, if we look to a country which has a non-Christian culture, and consider major studies in the last decade on psychiatric aftermath of abortion, we are led to conclude differently. In 1963, the Aichi survey reported that in Japan 73.1% of women who had been aborted felt 'anguish' about what they did. In 1964 Dr. Tatsuo Kasiki's report stated that 59% felt abortion was something 'very evil'.

This suggests that abortion cuts into a woman's nature, and that she will not remain psychologically unscarred after it. Freudian psychistrist obstetrician Julius Fogel, who himself has performed hundreds of abortions, wrote in the Los Angeles Times

I think every woman - whatever her age, background or

sexuality - has a trauma at destroying a pregnancy. A level of humanness is touched. It is totally beside the point whether or not you think a life is there. You cannot deny that something is being created, and that this creation is physically happening. Often the trauma may sink into the unconscious. But it is not as harmless and casual an event as many in the pro-abortion crowd insist. A psychological price is paid. It may be alienation, it may be a pushing away from human warmth, perhaps a hardening of the maternal instinct. Something happens on the deeper levels of a woman's consciousness when she destroys a pregnancy. [24]

Probably the best single study of the psychological aftermath of abortion is that of Eklbad's. [25] Eklbad interviewed 479 women prior to abortion and again 2½ to 3 years later. At the follow-up stage he found 10% felt the operation unpleasant, 14% had mild self-reproach and 11% had serious self-reproach and self-regret.

In the Swedish town of Malimo, Dr. P. Aren [26] studied 100 women who, having previously had a legal abortion, subsequently had a pregnancy, and gave birth to a child. He found that their reactions were as follows. 35% were content, 17% were content but had a 'bad conscience', 25% had mild guilt feelings and 23% severe guilt feelings. The guilt feelings were so severe in this last group that the women had suffered for varying lengths of time from nervous disorders, insomnia or decreased working capacity. Many of the women had been disturbed by the sight of small children. Abortion cannot therefore be considered as harmless from a psychiatric point of view.

Women are commonly amazed when the nature of the unborn child is described at its various stages. What would be the psychological aftermath of abortion if those gynaecologists who performed abortions freely were fully to inform their patients what exactly was being destroyed? I think many women would no longer wish to go through with an abortion. In practice, however, those promoting abortions indulge in euphemisms to hide what is actually involved. This is shown particularly well in the book *The Death Peddlers*. [27] A nurse, Henrietta Blackmon, gave advice on how best to counsel women about to have an abortion. If at all possible, the word 'abortion' is not to be used. Instead, the phrase 'a D and C' should be used, as these are so common. Blackmon argued that when speaking about the child her audience should 'use the word "foetus". This is a foetus; this is not a baby'." One should not say 'suck out' the baby, but rather, 'empty the uterus' or 'we will scrape the lining of the uterus'. Never should one say, 'we will scrape away the baby'. The reality of the action has to be diluted for consumption. This is made possible by the couching of all descriptions in clinical terms. Yet after an abortion by D and C it is factually true that what is left is a desmembered leg and an arm and a severed head, all of which could come only from a baby.

One situation which would seem to offer a compelling argument for abortion arises when a pregnant woman in a depressed state threatens suicide unless her child is aborted. There is a world of difference, however between a threat of suicide and actually carrying it out. In Birmingham, over a period of seven years, 119 women below the age of 50 committed suicide. Not one of these women was pregnant.[28] Suicide in the pregnant woman is extremely rare; in fact it is about one-sixteenth the rate seen in non-pregnant woman of the same age.[29] It is virtually impossible to ascertain accurately whether a woman is suicidal, and the woman who threatens suicide unless an abortion is allowed her obviously has a vested interest. On the other hand, abortion cane sometimes lead to suicide in women suffering guilt feelings as a result of having had an abortion. Russell Shaw, in his book *Abortion on Trial,* comments:

> The evidence on this point is inconclusive. It is at least worth reflection that the two highest suicide rates in the world for women in the 20-24 bracket are those of Japan (44.1% per 100,000) and Hungary (17.1% per 100,000) - two countries whose abortion rates are among the worlds highest. This has led Professor Shiden Inoue of Japan's Nauzan University to suggest a possible 'casual relationship' between abortion and suicide in these countries.[30]

'Every child a wanted child' is one popular slogan used to justify abortion. Everybody would agree that no unwanted child should be conceived. Yet the notion of 'unwanted' is

Cf. insert, p. 33.

difficult to determine. At what point of time is the child to be judged unwanted? At two months into the pregnancy, when the mother is vomiting and depressed, or perhaps on the day of delivery, when the mother has her child in her arms? In those circumstances where the child is genuinely unwanted by the mother, the rest of society takes over the support of and caring for the child. There is a long waiting list of would-be adopters brought about in part by the shortage of babies because of abortion.

It is also often suggested that unwanted pregnancies become battered children. Dr. Edward Lenoski, Professor of Pediatrics at the University of Southern California, for four and a half years made a study of 400 battered children. He determined that 90% of the battered children in his study were from planned pregnancies. There seems to be no simple relation between unplanned pregnancy and battered children.

The work of Forsman and Thuwe [31] is often quoted to show the dire consequences to the children born because an abortion has been refused. The authors studies the lives of 120 children whose mothers had asked for but had been refused an abortion on psychological grounds. The children were followed up to the age of 21, and compared with a group of children, born the same day, apparently wanted. In this study there was a higher incidence of anti-social behaviour such as criminal tendencies and drunkenness, among the group born to mothers who had been refused abortion. The study, however, is of at best limited value since the incidence of domestic tragedies in women refused abortions was compared with the incidence in women from stable home environments. The important comparison would have been with women granted an abortion. Dr. M. Sydney [32] has commented on this study that it is "misleading to compare children born following an abortion refusal with wanted children, because the hostile home environment which led to the abortion request is likely to leave the stigma mentioned. The control group in this case should be successfully aborted children". He went on to ask whether 100 aborted children could be considered better than 100 children with a marginally increased chance of being unfit for military service, needing psychiatric support or being registered for a

26

drunken offence.

These applications for abortions on psychiatric grounds took place in the years 1937 to 1941 however, and it was only in 1946 that abortion in Sweden was widened to include the mother's circumstances. Thus it seems unlikely that these women would have obtained a legal abortion in England in the pre-1967 Abortion Act era. This study should not then 'be used as a lever for abortion on request.'[33]

Nearly half the abortions performed in 1970-1 were on unmarried women. In the past, prospects for the unmarried mother and her illegitimate child have been bleak. They have been social outcasts, many of whom have had to rely on inadequate supplementary benefits which allowed them and their children to do little more than exist. It has usually been difficult for the unmarried mother to work, because of the problem of getting someone to mind the child. In any case, with the very low rates of pay for women, a mother would often be working for about £2 more than she would get in supplementary benefits, and so unless professionally qualified would be worse off working. A job would, however, provide the unmarried mother with much needed companionship. In the past where so many unmarried mothers have chosen not to work, the result has been that men have tended to think of them almost as prostitutes. It is not surprising, given these facts, that many single women have chosen to have an abortion. This has proved a false remedy, and has set back the improvement of the lot of the unmarried mother in society as a whole. At present the unmarried mother can earn £2 before it effects her supplementary benefits. Yet widows and wives of the disabled can earn £9.50 a week without effecting their benefits. This discrimination should be discontinued, and the unmarried mother given the same allowance as the widow.

Unmarried mothers with, say, one child, can claim a Family Income Supplement if they earn less than £21.00 per week. The supplement is one half the amount by which her income falls below £21.00. However, to earn this supplement the woman must work 30 or more hours a week. If the number of hours to be worked was reduced to 22 hours, many more unmarried mothers could benefit. The supplement's workings are to be reviewed in Autumn 1973. One hopes that some change is to be made.

In 1969 the Finer Committee on one parent families was set up. It is likely that it will make its report later this year. It is already known that one of its recommendations is that single families should receive a special social security benefit. The effects of such a benefit on the unmarried mother cannot be assessed at this stage, but will obviously be important.

At present the demand for pre-school play groups, day nurseries and other forms of day care outstrips supply, even when children of one parent families are given priority. It is to be hoped that the Finer Committee will also recommend increased financial support for the extension of these services.

Equal pay for women should also be something championed by those defending the life of the unborn child. The present affiliation orders are the subject of much hardship. Under such an order the putative father has to agree to pay the mother a certain amount each week, to be collected at the court. Apart from the inconvenience of the mother getting to the court, quite often she finds that there is no money waiting when she arrives, and there can be endless trouble as the husband's arrears mount up. It would be more sensible if the Department of Health and Social Security took over the payment of such orders, and made itself responsible for dealing with the father. The mother would then have a guaranteed source of income.

Each year about 20,000 children are adopted - ¾ of whom are illegitimate. It is not easy to give up your child for adoption. To wrap him up in a blanket and hand him over through the intermediary of a third party, to someone else must be one of the worse moments in a person's life and one never to be forgotten. Yet at least there is the comfort of knowing that in spite of everything you have tried to do your best for him. You have not destroyed him who was growing inside you.

It is gratifying that organisations such as Life, [34] which urges repeal of the 1967 Abortion Act, are also concerned to help women with a problem pregnancy. Life offer advice about finance, housing, social security and medical problems. It also offers unmarried mothers private accommodation during pregnancy. In Birmingham, Manchester and London, under a sister organisation called "Lifeline", they have opened a full-time office based on anti-abortion pregnancy advisory services. The Roman Catholic Bishop of Shrewsbury, Bishop Grasar, was in the news in mid 1973 for pledging the full resources of his diocese to help anyone with a problem pregnancy. This approach to the abortion problem is the only way - a tenderness for all life.

Chapter Four

Population

In January 1973 National Opinion Polls carried out a survey on behalf of the Birth Control Campaign Group. The survey, based on interviews with a sample of 1920 electors drawn from 100 constituencies in Great Britain, showed that 87% were worried about population growth, while a further 71% thought the government ought to do something about it. The ease with which public opinion has been made to panic over population must be one of the all time fascinating studies in the history of propaganda. The supposed population problem is often said to necessitate legalised abortion.

Our population growth is to be seen as the source of all evil. From it flow urbanisation of the countryside, over-crowding in terraces or on beaches, pollution, delinquency, mental illness and aggressive behaviour. In the atmosphere encouraged by such a vision it is not surprising that any means to cure the 'disease' of overpopulation are taken to be morally acceptable. Abortion is thus hailed as a necessary back-up for failed contraceptives. 'It would have been quite understandable', comments the Economist, 'if the demand for a population policy had gained momentum in the early 1960s. Then Britain was achieving a rate of natural increase of 355,000 a year. But natural increases for 1972 could be as low as 100,000. It has been almost ludicrous to watch the doomwatchers' case shrink in their hands, as estimates of Britain's population in the year 2,000 shrank from 74 million (the Government guess in 1965) to 63 million (the latest estimate released by Sir Keith Joseph last week August 1972).' [35]

In July 1973 the Central Statistical Offices once again said that at the turn of the century Britain's population would be lower than previously estimated. The new figure was likely to be 62.4 million, representing an increase in population of 6½ million by the year 2001.[36]

Since 1964, the peak year, Britain's birth rate has been falling by about 2% a year. This fall is due to the increasing number of women who go out to work, the wider use of contraceptive and, since 1967, the effects of the Abortion Act.

In 1971 there were 95,000 abortions on British residents and in 1972 115,000. An abortion performed is not, however, a reduction in births of one, for if a woman conceives, then has an abortion after three months, she is capable of becoming pregnant again during the time in which she would normally be bearing the child. Account has also to be taken of whether or not the persons having an abortion were using contraceptives, and the relative periods of sterility for abortion and child-bearing.

Taking all this into account, Hawthorn has calculated that in a non-contracepting population it takes approximately three abortions to reduce the number of births by one, and that, in a population using a 95% effective contraception, an abortion will prevent 0.877 of a birth.[37] Using these figures, then, abortions would seem to have reduced the number of births by about 60,000 in 1971 and 70,000 in 1972. This is to be viewed against an annual birth rate of around 900,000.

It is important to note that before the legalisation of abortion the birth rate was falling. Abortion has probably merely continued the decrease, though it is possible that, if abortion had not been made legal, there would have been a different public attitude towards the use of contraceptives or the use of abstinence, and that many conceptions would not have occurred to be aborted. Legalisation of abortion may have created its own clients, and cannot be considered as exercising its apparent demographic affect.

The argument that legalisation of abortion contributes to a diminution of the effective practice of contraception is supported by the study of Fredriksen and Brackett.[38] The Wynns have considered that the rising numbers of extra-marital conceptions, in spite of increased sales of contraceptives, is evidence that, 'unmarried women, unlike married women, are

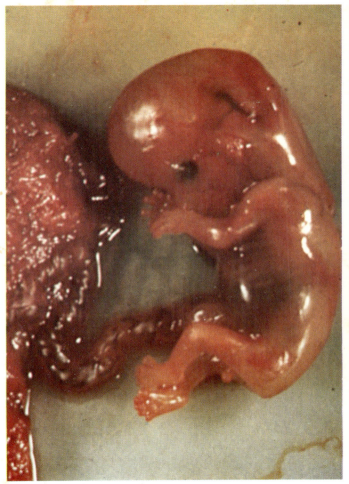

(From Handbook on Abortion)

Human Life at Eight Weeks

At this stage:
  — he (or she) will grab an instrument placed in his palm and hold on.
  — an electrocardiogram can be done.
  — he "swims freely in the amniotic fluid with a natural swimmer's stroke".

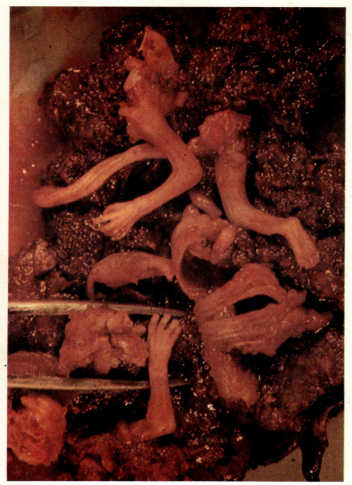

(From Handbook on Abortion)

Suction Abortion at 10 Weeks

Over one third of all abortions performed in the U.K. in 1971 were done by this method. It is like the D & C except that a powerful suction tube is inserted. This tears apart the body of the developing baby and his placenta, sucking the "products of pregnancy" into a jar. Sometimes the smaller body parts are recognizable as on this picture.

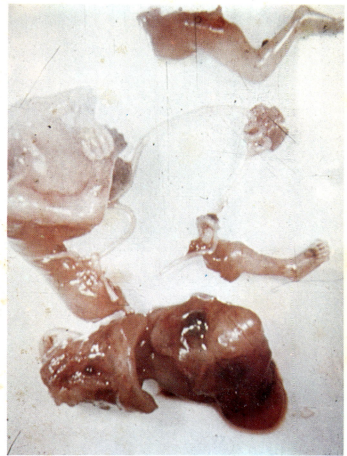

(From Handbook on Abortion, Photo by Dr. Wm. Hogan)

D & C Abortion at 12 Weeks

Performed between 7 and 12 weeks, this method utilizes a sharp curved knife. The uterus is approached through the vagina. The cervix (mouth of the womb) is stretched open. The surgeon then cuts the tiny body to pieces and cuts and scrapes the placenta from the inside walls of the uterus. Bleeding is usually profuse.

One of the jobs of the operating nurse is to reassemble the parts to be sure the uterus is empty, otherwise the mother will bleed or become infected.

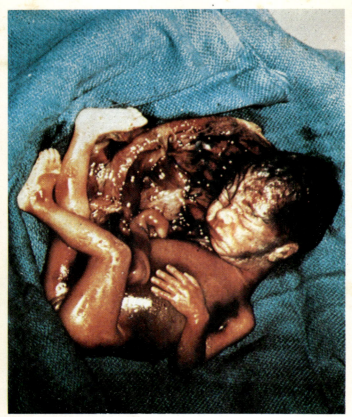

(From Handbook on Abortion)

Salt Poisoning Abortion at 19 Weeks

This method is done after 16 weeks when enough fluid has accumulated in the sac around the baby. A long needle is inserted through the mother's abdomen into the baby's sac and a solution of concentrated salt is injected. The baby breathes in and swallows the salt and is poisoned by it. The outer layer of skin is burned off by its corrosive effect. It takes over an hour to kill a baby by this method.

If the mother is fortunate and does not develop any complications she will go into labour and about one day later will deliver a baby such as the one above.

on the basis of three population models are 35,000, 48,000 or 70,000 acres a year. This loss has to be viewed against the total agricultural acreage of the United Kingdom, which is some 30 million acres excluding rough grazing. Evidence from the Ministry of Agriculture, Fisheries and Food indicates that increased agricultural productivity should more than compensate for urban expansion of the projected rates.[41]

It seems then ridiculous to suppose that Britain is in danger of becoming one vast concrete jungle. In New Scientist, (12 July 1973) it was estimated that it would take about 800 years at present rates of urbanisation completely to cover Britain with roads.

Overpopulation is also commonly held to be responsible for our pollution problem. The relation between pollution and population is however a very tenuous one. The USA, with a population density one sixteenth of ours, has far worse pollution problems than we do. Professor Barry Commoner has pointed out that over the period in which most of the USA's pollution problems either made their first appearance or became very much worse her population increase was 42% while her pollution increased by amounts varying between 200% and 53,000%. He concludes that the effect of population growth on pollution levels is very marginal and describes the birth control approach to pollution problem as, 'equivalent to attempting to save a leaking ship by lightening the load and forcing the passengers overboard. One is constrained to ask if there isn't something radically wrong with the ship.'[42]

A major cause of our pollution problems would seem to be the substitution of non-returnable cans for returnable bottles, of plastics for biologically degradable packaging, of detergents for soap and so forth. If industry were to devote a great proportion of its research budget to means of disposing of its waste this would go a long way to lessening pollution.

In certain respects pollution in this country has diminished while our pollution has increased. To quote Dr. Kenneth Mellanby, Director of Monks Wood Experimental Station,

The prospect of successful pollution control in Britain, even with a greatly increased population, are good if we are prepared to pay the cost in money and trouble. During the last 100 years the population has doubled, but in many ways our environment, particularly in our cities, has improved. The air of London is far less smoky, the Thames is no longer a stinking sewer.[43]

Population control then cannot be seen as the main answer to pollution.

High population densities are commonly asserted to be one of the chief causes of crime, mental breakdown, and illness caused by stress. The assertion is based on experiments in which large numbers of rats were put into cages and their behaviour observed. But there is no scientific validity in extrapolating from these experiments to human behaviour. Men, unlike rats, are gregarious, they chose to live in cities many years ago, and are used to doing so. As John Maddox argues, 'The belief that violence and war are accompaniments of overcrowding rests on the most shaky and disputed statistical basis. Who after all would think that the Netherlands, the most crowded of all the nations in Western Europe, is more given to violence than, say the United States.'[44]

In a study of contemporary population densities and human health, Factor and Waldron have concluded,

'careful studies on humans have failed to provide convincing evidence that contemporary population densities have significant harmful effects. There is no simple or reliable relationship between changes in population size and the frequency and intensity of wars. Brief exposures to extremely high densities have a variety of effects which are relatively small and not all harmful'.[45]

Further,

'it seems that, within, current ranges, density per se is not a significant cause of poor physiological health. Our study has not revealed convincing evidence of effects of population density on mental health and crime, but our methods have not been adequate to exclude this possibility. Although it would be of interest to explore further the relationship of density to other variables, it seems clear that public policy to improve health should focus directly on more well established problems such as poverty, malnutrition, inade-

36

quate education and health care.'

Even Dr. Paul Erhlich, a leading campaigner in the over-population movement, has admitted that, 'There is little relationship between the density of an area and the amount of crime or mental illness. When the economic levels of the areas are equated, density has no effect on juvenile delinquency.'[46]

The supposedly very limited natural resources are often quoted in justification for controlling population-growth in Britain. Typical of this attitude is the view of Mrs. Dilys Cossey, General Secretary of the Birth Control Campaign. 'The most important consideration therefore,' she states, 'is whether Britain's rate of population expansion is manageable in the context of world resources.'[47] However, there seems little fear that man will exhaust the mineral resources of the earth. Professor D.D. Hawkes, of the University of Aston, delivering his inaugural lecture as Professor of Geological Sciences, maintained not only that 17 million tons of material in the outer 10 miles of the earth's crust contain enough metal to meet all man's needs, provided he can extract it, but also that ores are still being formed. Professor Hawkes also took issue with estimates of current reserves. Based as they are on the limited data available which lists only known deposits of ore and which assumes no progress in mining or prospecting technology, they are 'always unreliable and invariably on the pessimistic side.'[48]

There is a tendency in the popular polemics on populations to regard resources as a fixed and finite quantity and not as a function of man's technological ingenuity and powers of discovery. This tendency is displayed in the well-publicised *Limits to Growth* by Professor Meadows, which used sophisticated computer models to arrive at a forecast of impending catastrophe. The use of sophisticated computer models suggests that the results are of a very precise nature and to be given great credence. But the validity of any computer calculation depends entirely on the data and the assumptions fed into it. Meadow's assumptions on the fixed and finite nature of resources are, then, 'a splendid example of how the supposedly objective Meadows's model turns out to contain a built-in bias in favour of collapse.'[49]

Boyle, however, writing in Nature, in September of this year, has said that the pollution crisis forecast by the Meadows' model can be "traced to a typographical error in the program. The corrected slightly revised model shows growth being limited before the year 2100 if the appropriate technology is introduced before the year 2000. Affluence without restrictive social policies is apparently attainable."

Britain cannot (thanks to scientific advances) be said to be suffering a great energy shortage. Indeed, it is possible that we might get close to energy self-sufficiency by the mid 80s.

'This prospect is possible because of the combination of a large coal industry, a major lead in nuclear technology and the oil and gas potential in the North Sea. With suitable planning and development of these resources a substantial degree of energy self-sufficiency in the mid-80s could be more than a possibility.' [50]

The survival of the human race in the past 500,000 years has depended on the continual improvement of man's scientific prowess. There seems to be no reason why this prowess should not continue to sustain him. Man's future is more threatened by the grim arguments of those who are so concerned about overpopulation than by the condition of world resources. The 'doomsday people' have invented a new social crime, that of having more than two children. It is distasteful to live in an atmosphere in which to have another child rather than a bigger house or bigger car can be looked upon as being socially irresponsible. Unwanted children, so the theory goes, should be aborted to help lessen the population problem. The theory, however, does not stop there. As Martin Ginsburg, a New York State Assemblyman who was crippled by polio incurred as an infant, and who uses metal crutches and hand and leg braces to move, observed in 1969 to the Assembly discussing abortion for the malformed unborn child, 'What this Bill says is that those who are malformed or abnormal have no reason to be part of our society. If we are prepared to say that a life should not come into this world malformed or abnormal, then tomorrow we should be prepared to say that a life already in this world which becomes malformed or abnormal should not be permitted to live.'

Talk of the 'quality of life' seems hollow when it is the quality of life of the chosen few that is really being considered.

Britain's likely population increases, according to the Government Report of the Population Panel (March 1973), are quite manageable in the context of this country; there is no need for the 'doomsday syndrome' from which so many people seem to suffer. The likely increases in population do not call for measures like abortion. It is unfortunate that the furore of the doomsday camp diverts attention from problems such as a greater distributive justice.

The population question in Britain is not merely a debate about the truth of certain facts, it is also a debate about values. The way in which 'value judgements' are unconsciously introduced is well displayed in the use made of the concept of 'optimum population'. Professor D.V. Glass, commenting on the concept of optimum population, made the point well when he said,

> 'there are some people undoubtedly who simply prefer birds to human people, therefore, they would have a much lower (human) population in this country and a larger area of nature reserves.'[51]

Because of the difficulties inherent in choosing which values are to be given priority the Government appointed Population Panel rejected the idea of an optimum population,

> 'there is no reason to suppose that it is possible to find a single criterion from which an optimum population can be deduced, nor is there any likelihood that the different criteria which might be proposed would point to anything like the same estimate of optimum population.'[52]

Many from the 'doomsday camp', - one thinks, say of Dr. Paul Erhlich - continue to talk of an optimum population for Britain. Despite the fact we already have 55 million people living in Britain, the figure mentioned is usually 30 million. This optimum they choose, not because the facts demand it, but because they lay great store by a primitive agricultural existence which will not damage the environment. They want to return to the villages of past centuries, untroubled by the pace and complexity of modern life. To achieve such a supposed paradise organisations such as the Conservation Society are prepared to press for taxes on families with more than the approved number of children. Abortion on demand would be a vital means in controlling population; euthanasia would also be acceptable. It would mean living in a society where the species was regarded as of prime importance, not the individual. The individual's right to live would be dependent on his age or his degree of physical perfection and where having children beyond a certain number would be an offence.

Chapter Five

The Results

In the first full year of the working of the Act there were 54819 abortions. The following year there were 86565 abortions. The number of abortions rose again in 1971 to 126744, and there was a further increase in 1972 to 156741. The 1972 figure corresponds to about 15% of all live births; taking into account the fact that 40,000 of the abortions in 1972 were to foreign visitors, abortion at present corresponds to about 11% of the number of live births. Abortion, then, is taking a large and still increasing number of pre-natal lives. One is entitled to ask for quite definite gains in return for the paying of such a price.

The claims of those who endorsed the 1967 Act taught one to expect, at the very least, a reduction in the number of illegal abortions, a reduction in the number of maternal deaths from abortion and a reduction in the illegitimacy rate. Has any of these things happened?

Before the Act was passed it was continually maintained that there were at least 100,000 illegal abortions a year. One arrived at this figure by looking at the number of admissions to hospitals for 'spontaneous and incomplete' abortions, and considering a proportion of these to have been criminally induced. One then multiplied the number arrived at by a factor of 3 or 4 because the illegal abortionist would presumably operate unsuccessfully in one of every three or four cases. The great difficulty with this method is in deciding exactly what proportion of patients had had an attempted illegal abortion. (The rate of spontaneous abortion has been estimated to be about 20% of all pregnancies, usually due to the foetus being defective.) Diggory,[53] reporting on 379 cases of abortion admitted to two hospitals on the periphery of London, concluded that about two thirds had probably been criminally induced, though patients often denied having done so. However, Bateman's study of women hospitalised in Lambeth led him to conclude that probably about 20% of cases were induced.[54] Stevenson's works in Northern Ireland led him however to conclude that the incidence of criminal abortion 'if it occurred at all in the series must be regarded as extremely rare'.[55] Of the patients admitted for 'spontaneous or incomplete abortion' one could with equal fairness consider almost none or perhaps one-fifth, or again perhaps two-thirds to have had an induced abortion. This variety makes the above method of estimating the number of illegal abortions meaningless. As the Lane Report says "we can find no satisfactory justification for this figure."

However, in 1969, C.B. Goodhart[56] estimated that there were not more than 20,000 criminal abortions per year. This he did by working on figures produced by Sir Dugald Baird in Aberdeen. Sir Dugald carried out a very liberal abortion policy in Aberdeen, performing 68 legal abortions per year between 1961 and 1963 for a population of 185,000. Baird believed that with his liberal abortion policy he had eliminated illegal abortions. On this basis Goodhart suggested a rate of not more than 20,000 per year for Britain as a whole. This figure seems much more well founded than the 100,000 that was commonly accepted during the passage of the Act. James has produced a dubious extension of Goodhart's work to arrive at a figure of at least 60,000 illegal abortions per year.[57] James pointed out that Aberdeen was an atypical area, in that it had a particularly good contraceptive service and therefore the number of conceptions would have been peculiarly low and the number of requests for abortion correspondingly smaller. It could just as well be argued, however, that a vigorous contraceptive campaign reinforces a mind set against pregnancy, and therefore artificially increases the number of requests for abortion. This is supported by the findings of International Planned Parenthood: 'Surveys in Korea, Taiwan and elsewhere have demonstrated that women who have used a contraceptive method such as the IUD are more likely than others to seek an abortion if they become pregnant because of either contraceptive failure or discontinuation of use.'[58]

James appears to have overlooked the fact that performing abortions fairly liberally in the local hospital is likely to make abortion appear more acceptable in the eyes of the local population. They would tend to request it more, despite the fact that they would not previously have considered a 'criminal' abortion. Baird was then probably performing abortions on more women than would have had illegal abortions. If we bear these points in mind, Goodhart's figure of 20,000 illegal abortions per year in the early 1960s could be seen as an upper limit.

In "Population Studies" July 1973 Goodhart used six independent lines of reasoning to estimate the extent of illegal abortion before 1968. Each of the six methods indicated that there were no more than 10,000 to 20,000 illegal abortion a year prior to the passage of the 1967 Abortion Act. Goodhart provides a rigorous defence of his earlier estimates based as they were on the Aberdeen data and on maternal mortality and finds that James's criticisms of his earlier work do not invalidate his conclusions. Goodhart points out that the death rate from legal abortion in 1969 was between 25.5 and 31.0 per 100,000. Now before the Act there were about 30 deaths a year from illegal abortion, if these referred to 100,000 illegal abortions, then it meant that it was as safe to have an abortion illegally before the Act as it was to have one legally after the Act. This is despite the fact that in Britain most illegal abortions are thought to be procurred by unqualified persons and often by the mother herself without assistance. It seems incredible that the legal and illegal death rates for abortion should be comparable. A "Lancet" article in 1969 had estimated that a criminal abortion before 1968 was ten times as risky as a legal abortion immediately after 1968. Using this then, the number of illegal abortions would only be about 10,000 before the Act. Goodhart even allows that at the extreme there could be twice as many deaths from illegal abortion than were in fact recorded as such. But even assuming this, the number of illegal abortions prior to the Act would still only be about 20,000. Goodhart also does a comparison of legitimate and illegitimate birth rates before 1968, together with what is known of the incidence of legal abortion.

He again concludes that the "true rate could not have exceeded 20,000 and was probably 15,000 a year" prior to the Act. Dr. Goodhart suggests that there will have been some transference from illegal to legal abortion and that possibly 4,000 to 9,000 illegal abortions a year have been avoided by the passage of the Act. The important point is that illegal abortion was far less prevalent than commonly accepted at the time of the passage of the Act and that it has by no means been eliminated. This is consonant with the experience of the German Democratic Republic, Yugoslavia, Hungary, Czechoslovakia, Japan, Switzerland, Bulgaria, Poland, USSR and Sweden. [59] It is possible that with abortion being made legal it appears less criminal to go to the back-street abortionist. The back-street abortionist may also have the added advantage of extra privacy.

It seems true that the 'legalisation' of abortion, whether locally, as in Aberdeen for many years, or nationally, as in Britain after 1967, creates its own clients. Gardner supports this thesis by referring to a Swedish study in which abortion was granted but not carried out. 'It was found that not more than 9% went on to provoke abortion, the other 91% although prepared to seek a legal one would not take illegal steps. This confirms the view that legal abortion is largely addressed to an entirely new clientele of women, who would never have had a criminal abortion and would give birth to the child if the possibility of legal abortion had not existed.'[60]

In its submission to the Lane Committee the RCOG rightly points out that, 'the number of cases of criminal and self-induced abortion in the past has been exaggerated.' They go on to point out that 'the total number of spontaneous and criminal abortions has not so far been materially reduced by the operation of the Abortion Act.'

The 1971 volume of the Report of the Hospital In-Patient Enquiry gives the following estimates for discharges from hospitals after treatment for spontaneous and incomplete abortions.

1965	71,800
1966	72,100

1967	69,900
1968	69,400
1969	67,400
1970	70,900
1971	65,000

If a large proportion of spontaneous and incomplete abortions are supposed to be criminal abortions, why has there not been a drastic reduction in the number of these hospital admissions since the Act?

The above figures suggest that if there had been 100,000 illegal abortions before the Act then there has not been any great reduction in their numbers since the act.'

The legalisation of abortion has then greatly increased the total number of induced abortions. The actual number of legal abortions performed is probably greater than that stated in the official returns. This is because, as the RCOG believes, 'considerable numbers of abortions in the private sector have not been notified to the Department.' [61]

Woman Detective Chief Inspector Brenda Reeve writing in the Police College Magazine this summer estimated that 'the actual number of abortions carried out by doctors is in fact twice the number quoted in the national statistics. These are effected both in the approved places and in surgeries, consulting rooms and other unlawful establishments.' This estimate was based on Inspector Reeve's experiences in Greater London where there are a large number of private clinics.

To pass on to the second claim made for the 1967 Act: has it reduced the number of maternal deaths from abortion?

The number of deaths from abortion of all kinds in England and Wales is in fact probably as high now as it was before the Act. [62] There were 29 deaths from abortion in 1967, the year before the introduction of the Abortion Act in 1968, and 29 deaths from abortion in 1969, the first full year after the passage of the Act (subsequent figures are still not available). This is despite the fact that there has been, significant improvement in the methods of treatment of the more serious complication of abortion.' [63] Any decrease in the number of deaths from criminal abortion is matched by a rise in the number of deaths from legally-induced abortion.

45

It is worth bearing in mind that deaths from abortion are and have been small compared with the number of deaths from other avoidable accidents, such as those in industry, in the home and on the roads. The important fact is, however, that the Abortion Act has not reduced this small number of deaths, which its supporters had claimed it would do.

The rate of illegitimate births has risen steadily from 31,000 in 1955 to almost 70,000 in 1967. By 1970 the number had dropped to 65,000. Assuming that, in the absence of the Abortion Act, the rate of increase of illegitimate births obtaining in the pre-1968 situation would have been continued into 1969 and 1970, then the real effect of the Abortion Act in 1970 was probably to reduce the number of illegitimate births by, - at the outside - about 10,000. But this reduction was obtained by performing over 45,000 abortions on unmarried women in 1970. This means that in 1970 there were about 35,000 extra conceptions amongst the unmarried. It would seem then that since the passage of the Abortion Act there has been a copulation explosion.

It is difficult to escape the conclusion that there is some relation between the passage of the Act and the increase in illegitimate conceptions. The increase in venereal disease rose from 3,500 cases of Gonorrhea in females in 1954, to 15,000 cases in 1969. Some 20% more female cases were reported in 1970 than in 1969, and in the first half of 1971 the increase was in the region of 40% on the 1969 figure.

The Act has reduced the number of illegitimate births by about 13%, but it has by no means produced the considerable reduction promised. And the reduction has only been obtained by taking about three times as many unborn lives again as the actual size of the reduction. The reduction has also to be set against the increased promiscuity and its companion, increased venereal disease, seemingly occasioned by the Act.

Probably the aspect of the Abortion Act that has most angered the general public is the great amount of money to be made from performing abortion in the private sector. This is particularly important, as in 1972 the fraction of abortions performed in the private sector had risen to just under two thirds. Mr. Joe Jordan, a Birmingham bynaecologist, was reported as having said at a public meeting that he was offered £12,500 a year for one half-day's work a week to do abortions. It is not surprising that gynaecologists in the private section operate what can only be called abortion on demand, since 99% of patients referred to them appear to have had their pregnancies terminated. [64] It is difficult to see how it can be in the interests of the women for the gynaecologists to have such vested interests in terminating the pregnancies that come to them. Women are unlikely to be made aware of the possibilities of side-effects from abortion, or of what alternatives to abortion there are. The RCOG itself believe that 'already there is evidence that those who see possibilities for financial gain by undertaking abortions are seeking to take up obstetrics and gynaecology', and that these young doctors are of 'inferior quality, so that the whole obstetrical and gynaecological service will deteriorate.'[65]

This is not only a frightening prospect in itself, but even more frightening when women with genuins gynaecological disorders may have their chances of obtaining a hospital bed lessened by the 'urgent' abortion cases. That this is indeed the case is argued by the RCOG in their Report on Unplanned Pregnancies:

> There is abundant evidence that the way in which the Act is working in practice is putting great strain upon both out-patients and in-patients services in the gynaecological departments of National Health Service Hospitals. These strains not only involve ethical and moral conflicts amongst doctors, nurses and para-medical staffs working in gynaecological wards, operating theatres and out-patients, but also effect the physical resources of departments and the service that can be made available to patients requesting consultation and treatment for the whole range of gynaecological disorders. [66]

The upshot of this is that many gynaecologists in the NHS find it 'quicker and easier merely to accede to a request without critical medical appraisal of the case.[67] This is to be contrasted with the attitude of one Liverpool gynaecologist, Mr. C.J. Moss, He says: 'I have taken recently to visiting patients in their own homes - and what I find so interesting is that the initial view that I formed about the advisability of termination changed radically when I saw them and their husbands in their own homes. In almost every case the initial decision that I would probably agree to termination has changed: after seeing them in their own home I have not agreed to do so. This simply supports the problem of devoting time to the patient.'[68]

The mother's best interests, then, do not appear to be at all served by the Act. It is not surprising that parliamentary opinion has moved steadily towards restricting the Abortion Law. Little more than a year after the Act came into operation, on 15 July 1969, Norman St-John Stevas' Bill to amend the Act was defeated by only 11 votes (210 against 199 in favour). In late 1970 Mr. Stevas put down an early day motion calling for an independent inquiry into the Abortion Law which would take into account the legal, social, ethical, medical and moral factors involved. It is interesting that over 260 MPs signed this motion, a considerable number of whom had in the first place voted for the present law but had had second thoughts. Others, while still ostensibly in favour, felt there was some need for clarification of the present situation. Finally, the present Conservative Government was forced to establish an enquiry, the Lane Committee. However, it completely ignores the early day motion supported by so many MPs in that it is related only to the working of the present law. This restriction is likely to hamper reform.

In 1972 Gallup conducted a survey to ask nurses their opinion of the Act. Of 682 hospital nurses who replied to a postal survey 73% thought that the interpretation of the Act had not been sufficiently strict. The result further showed that 69% thought legal abortion was being used as a method of birth control, and 7 out of 10 thought that other patients had had to wait for operations because of abortions.

On 30 April 1972 there was a mass rally in Liverpool against the present law. Estimates of the numbers varied, although the Guardian gave a figure of 40,000. 'It was,' it said, 'one of the biggest provincial demonstrations ever organised and was joined by contingents from all parts of the country.'[69]

The following year the Society for the Protection of Unborn Children [70] organised another demonstration, this time

48

in Manchester on 25 March. On this occasion, the Spectator reported, 'between 50,000 and 100,000 people turned up, and the mini counter-demonstration by the female chauvinist sows of Women's Liberation were quite dwarfed.' [71]

Politicians ignore the magnitude of these protests against the Abortion Act at their political peril.

Chapter Six

The Future

In recent years Rumania, Bulgaria and Czechoslovakia have put severe restrictions on their liberal abortion laws. In 1969 Rumania suddenly tightened its divorce and abortion laws to counteract an alarming drop in the birth rate. In 1973 Bulgaria, which used to permit abortion on demand, but where the birth rate was suffering much the same fate as in Rumania, changed its law so that abortion was forbidden for women who either have one or no children. The reason given was that between 25% and 30% of women suffer serious health hazards after abortion. In 1973 Czechoslovakia also tightened its abortion laws in order to stimulate population growth. It is interesting that while the Warsaw Pact countries discourage abortion the NATO countries encourage it. Liberal abortion Bills seem likely to be passed in West Germany and France in the near future, and Bills have been presented in both Italy and Holland. One wonders whether the unborn child is going to become a political football. Perhaps it will not be until the NATO countries become alarmed at how far they have fallen behind the Warsaw Pact countries that changes in Western European abortion laws will be affected. What is certain is that, the longer we have our liberal abortion law, the more we will become an 'abortion culture', with all its consequences.

In 1972 Dr. Hans Lohman produced a report on the psychiatric state of the Swedish nation. This was at the request of the Swedish Parliament, who had become alarmed at the increase in the number of people admitted to mental hospitals. Of the child's encounters with adults the report said, 'it is terrible to see the coldness with which (they) are confronted. Everywhere . . ., cold and without tenderness, with mouth clamped tight, silent and reproachful. What we have managed to put together for our children is an extremely cold and anti-child society.' Sweden has had legal abortion for 30 years. Now we ourselves seem destined to create another such anti-child society in Britain. If we are to avoid such a fate, the 1967 Abortion Act must be repealed or at the very least severely restricted. In doing so, we would not only be protecting the psychological environment of children, but also saving millions of unborn children from death. Already ¾ million babies have been legally destroyed since the Act.

It is often argued that laws against abortion are obsolete because they are ineffective. However, as shown in the previous chapter, the law that existed before the 1967 Abortion Act was successful, in that it contained illegal abortions to about 20,000 a year. This it did while permitting about 5,000 legal abortions a year to be performed on the NHS either because there was a danger to the life of the mother or because the mother's health was threatened with imminent, grave and lasting impairment. It is true though that the rich could go to Harley Street for a 'legal' abortion. The private sector for the rich was probably the source of another 10,000 abortions a year. This situation has to be contrasted with our present situation. There is no evidence of a decrease in the illegal trade, and legal abortions are now running at over 170,000 a year, whilst the private sector continues to make handsomely out of the situation, probably under-reporting the number performed, so as to avoid tax. The previous law against abortion was successful in keeping down the number of abortions probably not so much because of the deterrent effect of legal sanctions (these were rarely employed - there are only about 55 convictions for illegal abortions per year) but more because of the teaching effect of the law. For many, what is legal becomes what is moral. The law symbolised society's commitment to protecting the value of human life against deliberate or negligent afront. The law against abortion produced a situation which was, in Professor Finnis's words, 'indeed remote from the visible breakdown of the laws symbolic effectiveness under Prohibition.'[72] Finnis further comments that in countries where there are laws against abortion those persons wanting a much more permissive law have to agitate even to create the sense of a problem in the public mind, and people are shocked when they discover the supposed prevalence of illegal abortion.'[73]

A law against abortion similar to the one that obtained prior to the 1967 Act seems then a perfectly sensible objective. Whether repeal is a politically realistic possibility at the present time is debatable. Certainly, the Lane Committee itself was not able to consider the grounds on which abortion is permissible, but was merely empowered to investigate the working of the 1967 Abortion Act. At present two medical practitioners have to sign a certificate for an abortion to be legally performed. Might not one of the signatories to the certification permitting abortion be made that of an 'abortion referee', appointed by the Department of Health and not permitted to accept private fees? Then perhaps the lives of many unborn children would be saved. This referee might reveal that a mother's claim of grave injury to her mental health, is under the facts of a particular case, so trivial as to be sham in relation to the child's presumed desire to live. Fraudulent claims of rape or incest might be exposed. Fear of a gravely defective foetus might be shown to be unsubstantial by cross-examination of the physician proposing the abortion or by other evidence. It is possible that the inquiries of the 'abortion referee' might delay the performing of an abortion, with consequent increased risk to the mother's health; but there are other instances in which law has shown that it is able to devise techniques of accommodating itself to emergency circumstances - for example, the temporary restraining order.

If the actual grounds for abortion under the 1967 Abortion Act are to remain untouched, however, it is difficult to see how 'abortion referees' could consider much at all as evidence that a woman was not entitled by law to an abortion; the present law allows such an elastic interpretation.

It may be argued that Parliament's repeated intention before the passage of the 1967 Abortion Act was not to permit abortion on demand, and that it can, without altering the actual grounds for abortion in the Act, delete those sections that have been found to be inconsistent with this intention, notably S.1.(1). If the wording of the Act at this point were changed to: ". . . that the continuance of the pregnancy would involve serious risk to the life or grave injury to the health, whether physical or mental, of the pregnant woman," and the 'abortion referee' system instituted, this would act as a real defence for the unborn child. The Lane Committee have rejected the abortion referee system ostensibly because of the difficulty of finding people to appoint as referees. Perhaps it is really that such a system would interfere with their desire to see the private sector continue its work. A desire inconsistent with the Committies avowed condemnation of abortion on request.

The present law permits abortions up to 28 weeks. This gives rise to quite an anomalous situation, for within the same hospital an abortion can be performed on an unborn child of say, 24 weeks, whilst in a nearby ward doctors are fighting to save a baby of the same age born prematurely. Such doctors would have a 15% - 20% chance of success. The anomaly can be removed by making abortions legal only up to 20 weeks. Many countries, including Norway, Russia and Hungary, do not permit abortions past 12 weeks, unless it is to avert a danger to the woman's life or a serious risk to her health. The later an abortion is performed the greater the health risk to the woman. Reformers of the 1967 Abortion Act should be pressing for 20 weeks as the latest date at which an abortion is legally permissible, but they should also be at pains to point out that in view of the mother's increased health risk 12 weeks would really be the most sensible limit. In 1971 about ¼ of all abortions were performed after 12 weeks.

That London should now, be hailed the Abortion Capital of the World is again a matter of great public concern, yet the title has been well earned. In 1970 the number of abortions on foreign visitors was 10,603 rising to 32,000 in 1971 and 40,000 in 1972. This last figure is approximately one-quarter of the total number of terminations in that year. Most of these abortions were performed in the London area in private clinics.

It is a dubious honour to live in a country whose capital has the distinction of performing more abortions than any other in Western Europe. This could possibly be overcome by requiring that those seeking abortion possess a residence qualification.

In June 1973 the Law Commission recommended that a child born alive be given the legal right for proceedings to be initiated on its behalf against any person through whose negligence injuries were inflicted on it while it was in utero. This was a response to the problems the thalidomide children had in claiming for damages. If, however, a child can claim for negligence relating to a time when he was not yet born there must be a corresponding duty of care imposed on those guilty of the negligence. Under this recommendation, in other words, the law would confer a duty of caring for a human being held to have no legal rights under the 1967 Abortion Act! This contradiction could be resolved by admitting that the unborn child does have legal rights, and repealing the 1967 Abortion Act.

There have been many voices raised lately, notably in the House of Lords, in support of free supplies of contraceptives. They have argued that this would sharply reduce the number of abortions. However, the Government has enacted that, from 1 April 1974, there would be free advice for all from local doctors and contraceptives would be free of charge to women who had either had an abortion or a child within a year. Other persons, excepting those deemed to come into a social need category, would pay a prescription charge. Sir Keith Joseph expressed the view that 'there would be no sudden fall in abortions'[74] as a result of this policy. It is indeed by no means apparent that making contraceptives freely available will reduce the number of abortions. This as Wigfield's[75] study shows is because women taking the pill indulge in intercourse more often and with more partners than those not on the pill. The probability of conceiving is thereby increased. It is worth looking at the experience of Aberdeen in evaluating the merits of a free contraceptive service. Aberdeen introduced the first free service in Britain in 1967 and extended it to unmarried people in 1968. The figure for venereal disease rose from 751 in 1965 to 1,991 in 1972 (all ages), and from 98 to 457 in the 15-24 age group. Abortions on unmarried women increased from 32 in 1965 to 194 in 1970, and the number is still rising. (As pointed out earlier, Aberdeen has had a liberal abortion policy for about 30 years). It may be that if abortion continues to be easily available women will not bother to avail themselves of contraceptives. This might seem to go against the traumatic effects on women who undergo abortion mentioned earlier, which no one would want to undergo. Yet, as Gardner has pointed out 'in the whole Eastern block only in Poland has there been any success in persuading women to adopt contraceptive techniques instead of relying on abortion.'[76]

One would at least have hoped that the Family Planning Assocation would contribute to a change in the way abortion is regarded. Even this is not to be. Wigfield, a venereologist, aptly summarised the situation in a letter to The Times in April 1973. He wrote: 'Judging by some FPA pamphlets, publications and now cartoons, younger and still younger members of society are encouraged to believe that not only is it responsible to copulate without thought for a possible pregnancy but that premature sexual indulgence is expected of them. By a sin of omission this propaganda subverts the very fabric of society by ignoring love, marriage, personal responsibility and self-discipline in sexual relationships.'

It is interesting that the FPA has recently sent doctors in its clinics a leaflet from an abortion agency which advises anyone wanting an abortion that they can 'seek the help of your local Family Planning Association'.

It is distressing to see the Church of England stunned into silence on the abortion issue. So great has this silence been that in June 1973 Mr. Nicholas Fogg, of Christian Aid, initiated a letter signed by many other prominent Anglicans addressed to the Archbishop of Canterbury to the effect that the Church should be playing a much more active role in defending the unborn child. This would seem to be a clear Christian duty. The Christian Church from its earliest days has condemned abortion. In the Didache, or teaching of the twelve apostles, an authoritative statement of Christian principles composed in Syria not later than A.D. 100 and it may well have been written earlier, it is written:

> You shall not kill. You shall not commit adultery. You shall not corrupt boys, you shall not fornicate. You shall not practice medicine (in the sense in which a North American Indian medicine man makes medicine). You shall not slay the child by abortion. You shall not kill what is gene-

rated. You shall not desire your neighbours wife (Didache 2:2).

Other scriptural evidence of the early church's opposition to abortion is cited in Noonan's *Morality of Abortion*. It seems a pity that the Church of England does not seem to have seriously considered the words of the Protestant Professor Paul Ramsey of Princeton University: 'Until we are given a moral argument for abortion in certain sorts of cases that would not also be an argument for infanticide in the same sort of cases, then the proposed abortion is now morally the same as that for infanticide, even granting there is no tendency towards the production of the latter institution. Abortion would be (unless and until we are clearly shown otherwise) morally the same sort of "slaughter of the innocent". Those who believe this is the case have every right to say so." [77]

It is interesting that Christians such as Albert Schweitzer and Mother Teresa, both of whom have dedicated their lives to the service of the hungry, the unsightly and the poor, have positively rejected abortion. This suggests that the acceptance of abortion is a rejection of a tenderness for all life.

'Sex education' has been the source of much controversy in recent years. The phrase can mean little more than instruction in contraceptive technology, or it can really educate people in personal relations with sex as but an aspect. Ideally parents should be the ones to help the child integrate sex into his life, but unfortunately many are unwilling to do so. Yet today there are great pressures on the young, particularly from the media, to experiment and emulate adult behaviour. The examples portrayed do not encourage a more responsible approach by the adolescent. In the presence of pressures of such magnitude it falls to the school to assist the children's education in this field. It seems at the present time that almost all girls' schools have a programme of sex education, whilst boys schools seem to be lagging behind. This serves to illustrate the need to emphasise, that boys must be as responsible in sexual matters as girls. On the whole the course emanating from local authorities seem to cover all the topics one would wish to see covered, and are very well balanced. Much will obviously depend on the teachers. As the courses now stand, there is room for confidence that there will be an increase in happiness in human relations, together with a decrease in abortions and venereal disease.

However, problems raised in sex education are likely to increase in number and difficulty in the next few years. To the coming 'morning after' pill mentioned earlier, will probably be added the monthly pill, and an abortion pill. The monthly pill would be taken once a month and would produce the same external effect as an ordinary period, even if conception has occurred. It will in fact be producing an early abortion, and could even become the standard method of family planning. The abortion pill - a prostaglandin - could be taken anytime in the pregnancy to induce an abortion. These may even become available on prescription or purchased over the counter, provided a solution is found to the present side-effects. The practical consequences of these inventions needs proper consideration, For instance, most women will find it shattering to be faced with a 12-week-old unborn child, aborted because they decided in a moment of temper to take a pill.

The time is ripe for the 1967 Abortion Act to be restricted in the manner indicated in the previous pages. Those who are concerned to defend the life of the unborn child and to protect those members of society whom Hitler called 'useless eaters' must not grow weary of the whole disagreeable subject. They must lobby their MPs, write to their MPs, spend time informing themselves, possibly by joining SPUC or Life, or both, write to their local newspapers when relevant articles appear, offer positive help to women with problem pregnancies, sponsor suitable advertising campaigns. Good men must not remain silent: the stakes are as high as human life itself. I have tried to keep the tenor of this book calm and argue my case closely, but emotion does have a place. In essence the book is about whether the horrors shown in the illustrations to this book can be allowed to continue in a society that has pretensions to humanity. My answer is that only a pathetically sick society can allow such acts of barbarism to continue. Let's stop it now!

References

1. C.B. Goodhart, 1968 2 British Medical Journal 298
2. "Social trends No. 3" 1972
3. "International Planned Parenthood News," March 1972
4. Professor Goodhart, "Discussion" Biology and Ethics, pp 101, 103
5. M.G. Bulmer, *The Biology of Twinning in Man,* O.U.P.1970
6. Geraldine Flanagan, *The First Nine Months of Life.* Heinemann, p36
7. Leslie B. Arey, *Development Anatomy,* W.B. Saunders Co. 1954
8. J.W.J. Still, "Wash. Acad. Sci." 59:46 1969
9. D. Hooker, *The Prenatal Origin of Behaviour,* University of Kansas Press 1952
10. B.M. Patten, *Human Embryology,* 3rd Edition, Chapter 9, New York, 1968
11. *The Embryology of Behaviour,* Chapters 4 - 10, New York, Harper and Bros 1945
12. Petre-Quadrens et al. "Sleep in Pregnancy, evidence of foetal sleep characteristics", A.M.J. Obst. Gynaec 1967
13. Geraldine Flanagan, *The First Nine Months of Life,* Heinemann, p69
14. D.M. Rorvik, "Brave New World of the Unborn," Look, Nov. 4th 1969, p74
15. D. Callahan, *Abortion: the Law, choice and morality,* Macmillan, p365
16. In Ethics, Jan 1972, R. Gerber, "Abortion: Parameters for a decision", University of Chicago Press

18. Miss Barbara Smoker, Vice-Chairman of the British Humanists Association, letter to The Times, 22nd Jan. 1973

19. Address to the Royal College of Nursing by Sir John Peel, March 1972

20. R.F.R. Gardner, *Abortion the Personal Dilemma,* Paternoster Press, p66

21. Stallworthy, "Legal Abortion: a critical assessment of its risks," The Lancet, December 1971

22. Dr. Margaret and Arthur Wynn, "Some consequences of induced abortion to children born subsequently", (Foundation for Education and Research into Child-bearing)

23. Ibid

24. Los Angeles Times, 7th March 1971

25. M. Eklbad, "Induced Abortion on Psychiatric Grounds: a follow up study of 479 women." Acta Psychiat. Neural Scand. Suppl 99:238, 1955

26. P. Aren, "On legal abortion in Sweden: tentative evaluation of justification of frequency during the last decade." Acta Obstet et Gynec. Scand. Suppl 1, 1958

27. Paul Marx, *The Death Peddlers,* St. Johns University Press, p21

28. M. Simm, "Abortion and the Psychiatrists", B.M.J., 1963, 2, 145

29. A.J. Rosenburg et al, "Suicide, Psychiatrists and Therapeutic Abortion", Calif. Med. 102:407, 1965

30. Russell Shaw, *Abortion on Trial,* Robert Hale

31. H. Forssman and Inga Thuwe, "120 Children after application for therapeutic abortion refused," Acta Psychiatrica Scand. 1966, 42, 71

32. Dr. M. Sydney, Letter to The Times, March 1972

33. R.F.R. Gardner, *Abortion: the Personal Dilemma,* Paternoster Press, p227

34. Life, 35 Kenilworth Road, Leamington Spa, Warwickshire. Lifeline, London, Tel. 01-222 6392

35. The Economist, August 1972

36. The Times, July 11th 1973

37. Geoffrey Hawthorn, "Population Policy: a modern delu-

sion," Fabian tract 418

38. H. Frederiksen and J. Brackett (1968) II, The Lancet 167, 168

39. J. Maddox, Nature, Vol.234, December 31st 1971

40. Report of the Population Panel, March 1973, p3

41. Ibid

42. Barry Commoner, *The Closing Circle,* London 1971, Cape

43. *The Optimum Population for Britain,* Academic Press

44. John Maddox, *The Doomsday Syndrome,* Macmillan, p5

45. Factor and Waldron, "Contemporary Population Densities and Human Health," Nature, Vol. 243, 15th June 1973

46. Journal of Applied Psychology, Vol.1, 1971

47. Mrs. Dilys Cossey, Letter to The Times, 15th August 1972

48. Prof. D. Hawkes, Nature, Vol.242, 16th March 1973

49. Nature, Vol.242, 16th March 1973

50. National Coal Board Chairman, The Times, 18th May 1973

51. Prof. D.V. Glass, 1st Report of the Select Committee on Science and Technology, p208, para 775.

52. Report of the Population Panel, March 1973, para 383

53. P. Diggory, Abortion in Britain: proceedings of a conference on abortion held by Family Planning Association 22nd April 1966, Pitman

54. D. Bateman, "Cases of Abortion Treated at Lambeth Hospital 1960 - 1967" J. Obstet. Gynaec. Brit. Commonw. 75:1169 - 72 (1968)

55. A.C. Stevenson et al, Annals of Human Genetics, p395, 1958 - 59

56. C.B. Goodhart "Estimation of Illegal Abortion", Journal of Biosocial Sciences, 1969 I 235.

57. W. James, *Population Studies,* 1971, p327

58. International Planned Parenthood News, March 1972

59. *Induced Abortion:* a documented report by Thomas W. Hilgers MD, p52, Minnesota Citizens Concerned for Life Inc., Southeastern Regional Office, Box 744,

60. R.F.R. Gardner, *Abortion the Personal Dilemma,* Paternoster Press, p63

61. Report of the Royal College of Obstetricians and Gynaecologists to the Lane Commission, p3
62. Report of Confidential enquiries into Maternal Death in England and Wales 1967 - 1969. Report on Health and Social Subjects No.6, London H.M.S.O. 1972
63. Report of RCOG on Unplanned Pregnancy, p21
64. Ibid, p48
65. Report of RCOG to Lane Commission, p14
66. RCOG Report on Unplanned Pregnancy, p87
67. RCOG Report to Lane Commission, p6
68. "The Abortion Act 1967", p89 by Med. Pract. Soc.
69. The Guardian, 1st May 1972
70. Society for the Protection of Unborn Children, Hon. Sec., 47 Eaton Place, London SW1X 8DE
71. The Spectator, 31st March 1973
72. Prof. J.M. Finnis in "The Morality of Abortion: legal and historical perspectives", edited by John Noonan, p185, Harvard University Press
73. Ibid
74. The Times, 27th March 1973
75. Wigfield A.S. (1970) British Medical Journal 4 342-345
76. R.F.R. Gardner, *Abortion the Personal Dilemma,* Paternoster Press, p38
77. Prof. Paul Ramsey in "The Morality of Abortion: legal and historical perspectives", edited by John Noonan, p86, Harvard University Press